Weight Loss Revolutionized

Burn Fat Easily

Table of Contents

These are some of my other books below, and my website is
www.LosingBellyFatMission.com :

https://www.amazon.com/dp/B06XB4WHZX
http://www.amazon.com/dp/B06X9LXBB8
http://www.amazon.com/dp/B06WLK7497
http://www.amazon.com/dp/B06W54JKQN
http://www.amazon.com/dp/B06X6DJ9K3
http://www.amazon.com/dp/B06WGNJ9N3
http://www.amazon.com/dp/B06W549TBD
http://www.amazon.com/dp/B06VTF5DQJ
http://www.amazon.com/dp/B06WRPSBKK
http://www.amazon.com/dp/B06WD194JR
http://www.amazon.com/dp/B06WCZTK7Y
http://www.amazon.com/dp/B06X3QN1HT
http://www.amazon.com/dp/B01N19WBF2
http://www.amazon.com/dp/B01N2AVECA
http://www.amazon.com/dp/B01N4VZIAV
http://www.amazon.com/dp/B00QJJFS1C
http://www.amazon.com/dp/B01EMNO2MW
http://www.amazon.com/dp/B00SSFWCPA
http://www.amazon.com/dp/1520531230
http://www.amazon.com/dp/B01N4V7SR9
http://www.amazon.com/dp/B00SX58DUI
http://www.amazon.com/dp/B010K7YP62
http://www.amazon.com/dp/B012LAYNNQ
http://www.amazon.com/dp/B00RVX3KY2
http://www.amazon.com/dp/B01MR6SWGW

http://www.amazon.com/dp/B00XF6G4HO
http://www.amazon.com/dp/B01F1472N2
http://www.amazon.com/dp/B00PQ0TUPU
http://www.amazon.com/dp/B00PP8OZJ4
http://www.amazon.com/dp/B00QH7DY4Y
http://www.amazon.com/dp/B01052010G
http://www.amazon.com/dp/B00QDHXN7Q
http://www.amazon.com/dp/B00PO0IQIO

Among others.

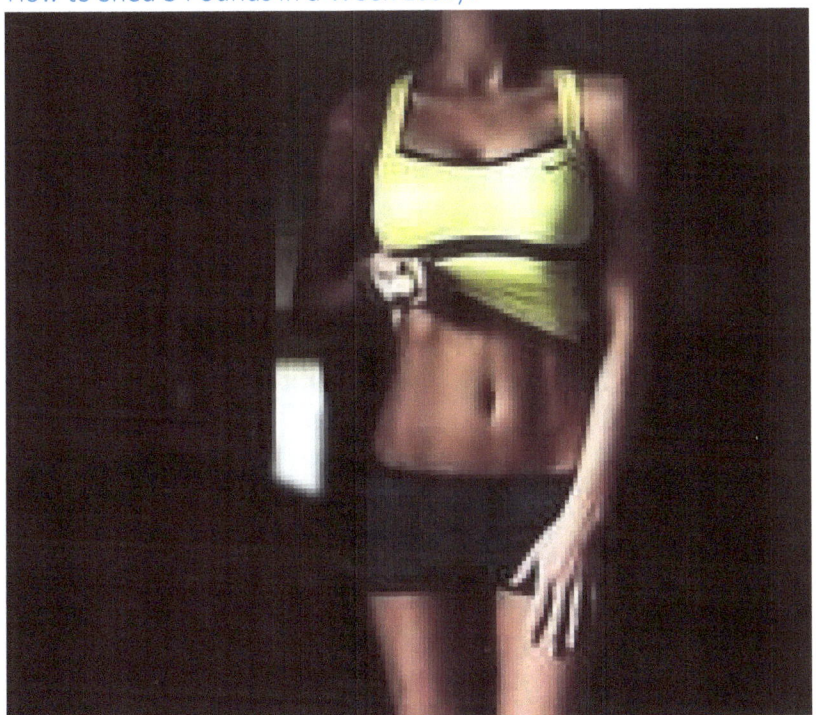

If you want to know how to shed 5 pounds in a week then you are reading the right article! Losing weight is all about giving your body what it needs and when it needs it. If you rush to lose weight chances are you will gain it all back. So I wanted to write an article that really shows you how to lose weight fast and in a manner where it will not come back. That's when I came up with a little strategy that seems to work really well. Basically you will need to gradually work your way into this program over a course of 7 days. I know that may seem hard to gradually work your way into the program when you only have 7 days but it is all perspective.

So let's take a look below on what you need to know when it comes to learning how to shed 5 pounds in a week.

- Day 1 you need to stop eating all junk food and start eating fresh fruits, vegetables and lean meats. You also need to walk a mile on day one. Do very light weight lifting if you are a female and moderate lifting if you are a male.

- Day 2 you need walk one mile and cut your calories in half. Make sure that you are still eating healthy foods though and no junk foods at all.

- Day 3 you need to start running 1.5 miles. Keep your calorie intake at half of what you were eating when you first started the program. Again do light weight lifting if you are a female and moderate lifting if you are a male.

- Day 4 you need to walk around two miles. Your calorie intake should now lower to 40% of when you first started on day one.

- Day 5 you need to walk at least 2 miles. Still eat around 40% of the calories you were eating when you first started the program. Again you need to lift light to moderate depending on your gender.

- Day 6 you need to walk 2-3 miles and keep your calorie intake at 40%. Of course continue to eat healthy also.

- Day 7 you need to walk 2-3 miles and keep your calorie intake at 40%. Do your light lifting session and continue to eat healthy. That's all there is to it!

You will lose 5 pounds for sure following this simple little diet and exercise plan. It's really not hard to lose 5 pounds in a week or even 10. Of course before trying this program I suggest you talk to your doctor first just to make sure your body can handle a change like this. Also remember if you want to lose more weight be sure to check below for a full detailed program. I wish you good luck on learning how to shed 5 pounds in a week!

The 5 Simple Rules To Follow To Transform Your Body Like Never Before In 30 Days Or Less!

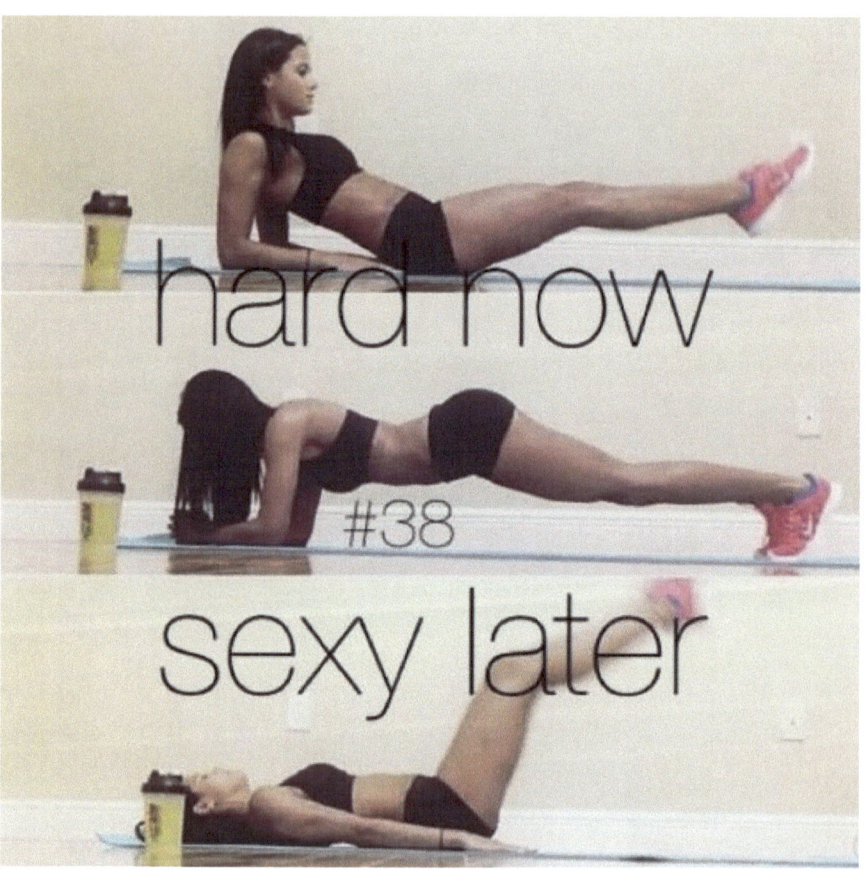

Do you want to be able to transform your body in 30 days or less? If so, then in this article you are about to discover 5 rules that I followed that easily had me drop pounds of fat like never before! Take a quick break from your hectic day and read on to learn more... The Build Muscle Rule... First off, building lean muscle is by far the most important type of exercise you have to do in regards to burning off fat and losing weight. Many people think it is cardio.

Although cardio is very important, building muscle has A LOT more benefits! You'll increase your metabolism and you'll burn off calories of fat AFTER you are done your workout (even 24 hours after)... to name just a couple of benefits! Secondly, please understand that you DO NOT have to get gigantic muscles! You simply need to build lean muscle. Thirdly, the best type of resistance training I recommend is anything that works multiple muscle groups at once. This would be either/or body-weight exercise routines or compound weight training such as bench presses or squats.

The Cardio Rule... For cardio, the best thing I recommend is anything that will skyrocket your metabolism. The 2 best types of cardio I recommend for this is H.I.I.T (high intensity interval training) or normal high intensity training. An example for H.I.I.T is to do something like jogging for 2 minutes and then sprint as fast as you can for 30 seconds, and then repeat both for up to 20 minutes for a killer workout! An example of a high intensity workout could be circuit training using body-weight exercises or even something such as sprinting or high knee skipping. The benefits of higher intensity cardio is that it's a faster workout, it's more fun to do, you MAINTAIN muscle tissue with these exercises, you'll get results much faster, and so much more!

The What You Drink Throughout The Day Rule... What you drink plays a significant role in either helping you lose weight and body fat... OR... putting on weight and body fat. What I recommend you avoid is excessive alcohol, excessive caffeine, ALL TYPES of soda, and ALL TYPES of sugary fruit juices. What I recommend you do drink is plenty of fresh water (of course!), all types of teas (which has plenty of antioxidants in them), apple cider vinegar (3 tablespoons mixed into 8 ounces of water, and have this 3 times a day for AMAZING health benefits), a moderate amount of coffee (without all the extra calories), and all natural FRESHLY made fruit and/or vegetable juices (with NOTHING added).

The Most Forgotten Rule... GO TO BED! The Ultimate Rule That Gets You Slimmer In The Next Couple Of Weeks... Go on a diet that mixes the most effective types of foods with a system guaranteed to skyrocket your metabolism to the highest peak. This type of diet is something I went on and I ended up losing as much as 25 pounds in a month... NATURALLY!

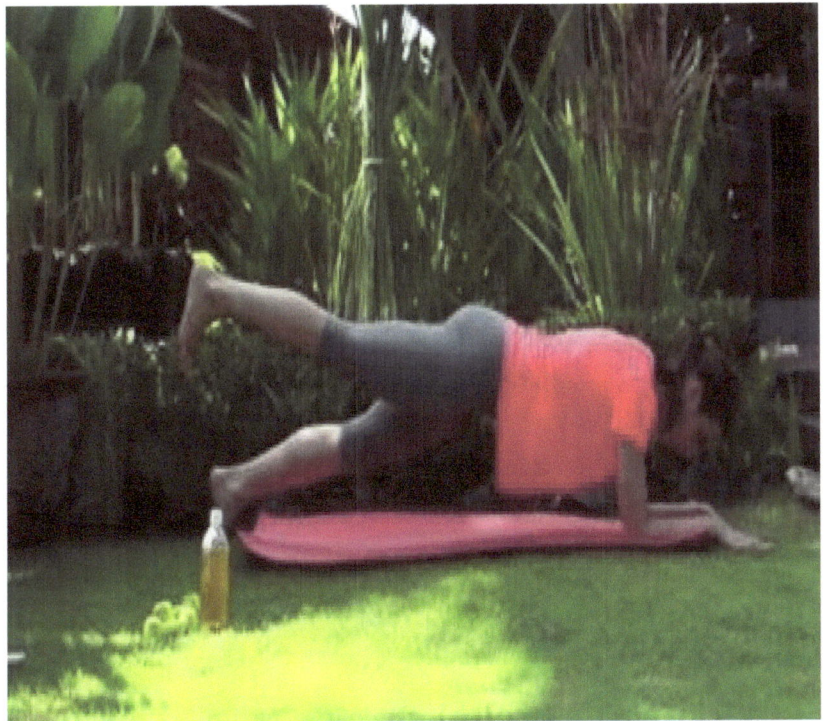

Metabolism is a series of chemical reactions that that determines the rate of how one's body produce and consume energy to support a their everyday activities. Having a high metabolism rate will enables you to burn fat more and lose weight faster with the least possible activity, and this is the dream of every one who is losing weight or trying to lose weight to get fit and lean.

Several factors are involved in determining the metabolism rate. It defers from one to another, but there are some factors that will actually affect every body's metabolism rate. In the up coming paragraphs we will discuss come of the most effective factors that could affect your metabolism greatly. Generally, the more the muscle you have the more the energy you need the more your body will burn fat for that.

So the key for that all is to have a lean fit body, and you could achieve that by exercise. You had to make some time in your busy schedule for work out, at least twice a week for at least 30 minutes. This should be a routine, a useful habit, try to make it fun so you would never leave it, and also put into your consideration that this is very important for your health.

Food, it is one of the most important factors as it determines the amount of energy which will be taken by our bodies. So here we will discuss some simple rules for your eating habits. First of all don't skip breakfast, a lot of people who do so are overweight or obese, and most of the people who take breakfast are the fit ones. It was proven that breakfast is the most important meal of the day. Metabolism rate increases dramatically if you ate your breakfast in the early morning, but if you waited to the afternoon or till mid-morning it will decreases.

Try to increase the water intake. Our bodies are nearly 70% water, so it is very important for us. Also, metabolism cannot be done without water. Also water clean our bodies from toxins, a healthy body will has a higher metabolism rate. Avoid eating much sugar, as sugar enables the body to store fat.

Try to make your meals smaller in quantities and increase the number or meals; it is advisable to eat 4 to 6 small meals than to eat 2 to 3 bigger ones. Also try not to skip any meal, as this will maintain the metabolism rate at a higher level. Beside exercise to build a fit body and planning your meals to healthier ones, there are some factors that also affect the metabolism rate.

Sleeping for at least 7 hours a day will be the best you can do for your body after a long day of activity. Also, muscles are built in the last couple of hours of deep sleep. Keep yourself away from stress. As when people are stressed their bodies release cortisol which will decreases the rate of metabolism, also stressed people eats more. At last those are some metabolism boosters to aid you through your journey to lose more weight.

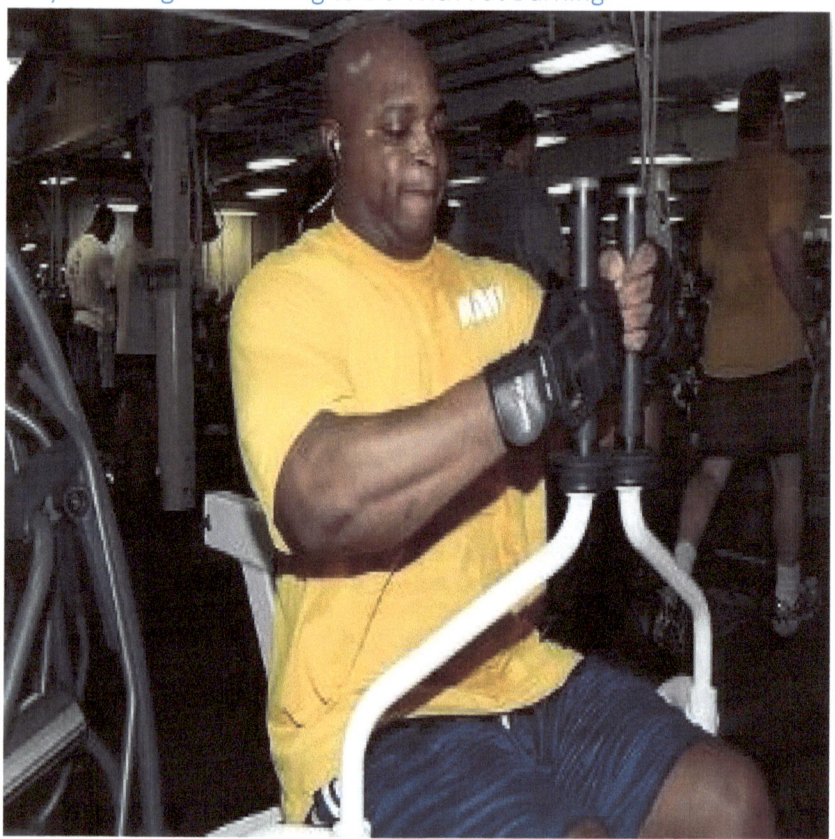

When we decide that we need to lose some weight, the first thing that comes up to my mind may be start working out. What kind of exercise that helps us lose weight the most? The recommendations from people around us are usually get a private training session with personal trainer A at gym B or personal trainer C at gym D. Since most people will recommend a gym as the best place to burn fat fast, we sign up for a gym membership.

The first time you get into the gym, you may be overwhelmed by all the devices and exercises. A guy is doing presses, another guy is running on a treadmill, and there are a bunch of people jumping up and down in body pump class, RPM class, etc. Since you are not familiar with all those exercises, you may have started with the simplest exercise, running on a treadmill. The theory is, sweat more and you will burn fat. Run faster and you are going to burn more calories. The more calories you burn, the faster you are going to lose weight. Isn't weight loss as simple as calories in minus calories out? If we eat very little and sweat a lot today, we are going to lose weight eventually, aren't we? Unfortunately, it's not as easy as said.

Most people fail to lose their weight simply by eating less and sweating. As a matter of fact, we do know that eating rice, bread, or any other sources of carbohydrate will give us energy to live. We also know that not we will feel the lack of energy if we don't consume carbohydrates. We come up with a conclusion that carbohydrates are the main source of energy. Despite the fact, people still think that the only way to burn fat is by exercising. How on earth will your body burn fat if its main source of energy is carbohydrates? The faster you run on a treadmill, the more likely that the calories burned comes from carbohydrates, not fat.

Fat is the source of energy when we work out in moderate intensity. When a person runs really fast, his body needs explosive energy which it can only get from carbohydrates. The multi-step process of breaking down fat into energy takes too much time that it cannot be used as a source of energy in a high intensity workout.

The best way to burn fat is by exercising in moderate intensity, when your heart rate is above 65% of its maximum heart rate. Two hundred and twenty minus your age is your estimated maximum heart rate. If you are 25, then you are going to have to keep your heart rate around 127 beats per minute. The easiest way to monitor your heart rate is by wearing a heart rate monitor, but you can also calculate your heart rate by counting your heart beats for 10 seconds and multiply it by 6.

What about weight training? Can it help us lose weight? During weight exercises, your body most likely uses carbohydrates as its source of energy due to the reason explained above. Nevertheless, you can do weight exercises for around 45 minutes and force your body to use up all its carbohydrates. When it has used up all the carbohydrates, this is the time to run on a treadmill or do other aerobic exercises and keep your heart rate around 65%-70% of your maximum heart rate.

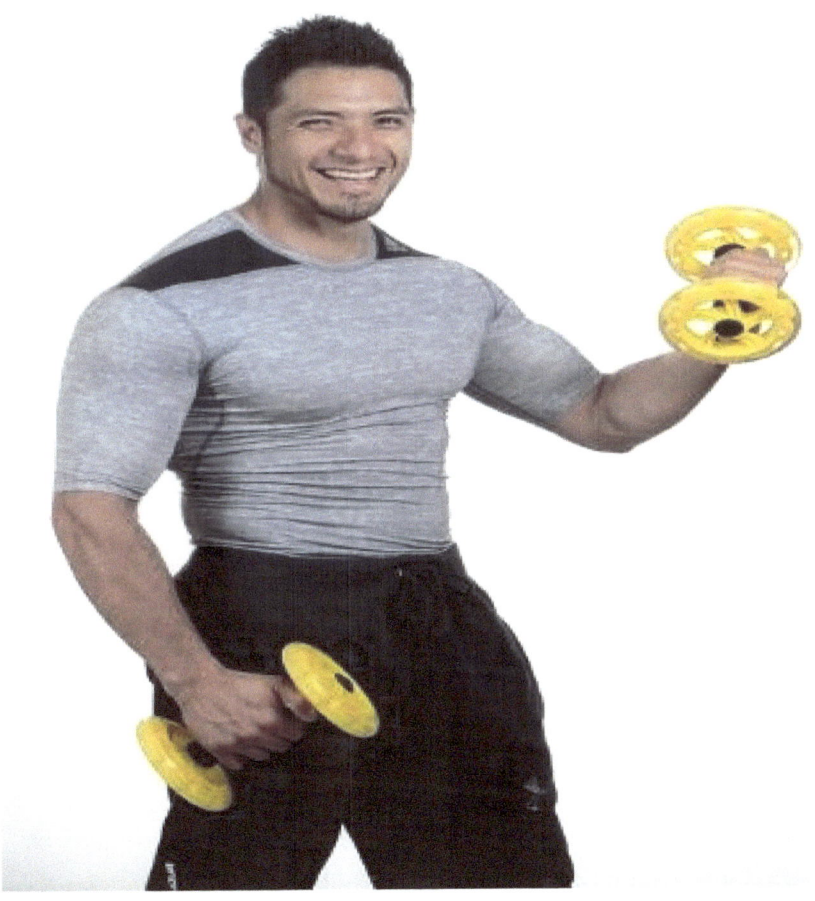

Having a beer belly, pot belly or love handles is one thing that nobody wants. Having excess fat around your mid section is not only unsightly but can also put you at risk of heart disease, high blood pressure and various other health related problems. The good news is that it is very simple to get rid of your extra gut, but unfortunately the simple steps are hidden amongst phony weight lost pills, products and courses. Leaving people confused and disappointed and no closer to losing to reaching their goals.

In this article I'm going to show you how to lose your excess fat, using a few steps that are easy to apply. I will be honest with you though, and tell you now that I can show you these simple steps, but it is up to you to implement them and stick with them, so you will need to be determined and show good will power! That said once you start seeing some results, weight loss will soon stop becoming a chore and may even become fun! Something else that I should mention is that you can't spot reduce fat, it is impossible to remove fat from just one spot on your body.

When you start losing weight you may find that fat does go from some location on your body faster than others, but eventually even your stubborn spots, i.e. your belly, will start to disappear as well. I would also like to dispel the myth that abdominal exercises such as crunches and sit ups will get rid of your stomach fat, all this really does is tone the stomach muscles underneath the fat. This will make your stomach look great, but only once you get rid of the fat that's hiding those muscles.

I won't keep you waiting any longer, let's move onto the steps you need to take to get rid of that belly fat. I have broken these down into two parts, these are diet and exercise. Diet: Firstly don't be put off by the word diet. Most people associate dieting with starvation, if you diet properly this isn't the case at all. There are a few simple changes that you can make which will help to get rid of that big belly very quickly.

The first change that you need to make is to stop eating processed and junk food and start eating natural nutritious foods. Processed foods are full of artificial additives, hydrogenated or trans fats and refined sugars. These are very bad, that have the ability to pile on fat and they contain no nutrition for your body, in fact they are that bad they can even extract nutrients from your body! Getting rid of these types of foods will bring you amazing results, many people underestimate how powerful it is when you are trying to lose weight. You should replace all this processed junk food with natural fibre rich vegetables, fruits, wholegrains and lean meats. The fruits and vegetables will supply your body with the nutrition that it needs to function at its most efficient level, this means that it will be a lot easier to burn off body fat. Going for the wholegrain versions of rice, pasta and bread are a lot better than their white alternatives which are full of refined carbs which are as bad as fat! These wholegrain foods should however still be limited in our diets.

Lean meats such as beef, chicken and fish are great sources of protein, this will help to prevent the breakdown of muscle when losing weight. The next change that you should make to your diet is to eat more often and reduce your portion size. This may sound odd, but let me explain. Your body can only successfully process a certain amount of food in one sitting, the rest will just turn straight to fat. The best tactic for losing your belly is to actually eat six smaller meals each day, rather than two or three large ones. Eat more often will actually increase your metabolism, which makes it easier for you to lose weight. It also feeds your body with a constant supply of the nutrients that it needs, keep your energy up throughout the day and prevent craving and binges. If you make those simple changes to your diet today, you will be well on your way to shedding that excess fat from your waistline. We're not done there though, let's move on to the next thing you need, which is exercise.

Exercise: Exercising is very important to successfully and permanently losing that belly fat. Regular cardio workouts are great for burning off fat. If you have never really exercised before you can start by walking for at least thirty minutes three times a week, then move onto more challenging exercise such as jogging, cycling or rowing. You can increase the length of your workouts and also add in more each week, three or four per week is great though. If you can't bear the thought of this type of workout, then I suggest you find an activity which gets your heart rate up that you enjoy doing. Maybe playing tennis, football or roller skating three or four times a week; these aren't as effective at burning fat as the cardio workouts we mentioned, but they are still great.

The next thing that you should start doing to improve your fat loss is to include two to three resistance training workouts into your weekly routine. A good weight lifting workout is not only a great fat burning workout, but it also will help you to add lean muscle to your body. This will not only make you look great and feel firmer once the fat is gone, but also muscle actually burns up calories just by being there, how great is that!

A lot of people worry about training with weights because they are worried about becoming muscle bound, but you really don't need to worry about this. Building large amounts of muscle is a lot harder than you think, the right type of training, overeating of calories and correct protein consumption are all required to build a lot of muscle, along with a few other things. If you are trying to lose weight you are only likely to put on a small amount of muscle, but that is all you need to gain the benefits that we have already mentioned. So that it is, as you can see it does take some work but it is very simple to apply these tips. If you apply them today you will start seeing your belly fat starting to shrink very quickly!

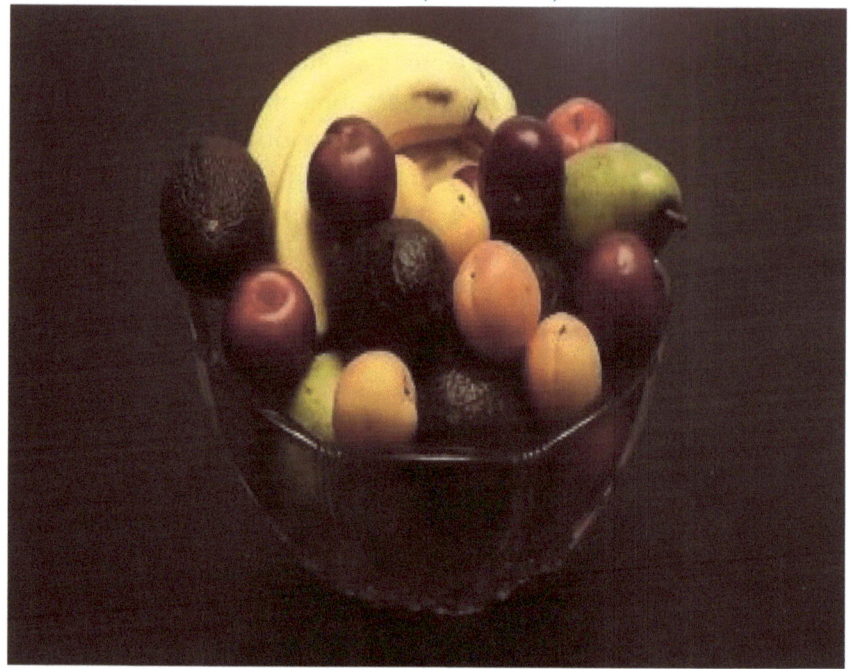

Obesity is a dangerous problem to have if not kept in check. It not only shortens your lifetime but also seeks to worsen the quality of life as well. If you are also one of the millions who are battling obesity, take just a quick 5 minutes out of your busy schedule to read this article and find out powerful tips that will help you burn fat and lose pounds quickly, safely, and easily!

1. Prepare a drink of lemon juice, honey and ginger mixed with water, and drink it whenever hungry to detoxify your body. You feel good, no shortage of energy, no cramps, nothing. Definitely, it will help you to lose pounds quickly.

2. Include plenty of raw vegetables, eggs, lean beef, fish and some fruits (generally oranges and apples). Your new way of eating should be like this: half the plate of vegetables except potato, one forth of the plate - fish or white beef, and the rest may be fruit. Avoid bananas because they're too starchy and sweet.

3. Start to take breakfast and stop eating just prior to sleeping. Breakfast will improve your metabolism and help you to burn calories quicker, although you never think it may be so significant for lose pounds quickly. You should take plenty of water in a day. Water does not let you hungry, cleanses your body and increase metabolic rate.

4. Distribute your daily calorie intake throughout the day and begin to eat four to five times each day, having lighter meals.

5. Rather than drinking juice, eat fresh fruits. Juice is not good for weight reduction. If you feel thirst, drink some water instead of juice.

6. Keep yourself motivated and full of activity whole day. I'm of the opinion that when you are busy, you don't have any time to eat. This works like miracle.

7. Avoid sweets and fried foods. If you want to eat something unhealthy, move those meals to the morning because metabolism is faster in the morning compared to the evening. If you follow this plan faithfully, it may appear too easy to lose pounds quickly and safely.

These are some of my other books below, and my website is
www.LosingBellyFatMission.com :

https://www.amazon.com/dp/B06XB4WHZX
http://www.amazon.com/dp/B06X9LXBB8
http://www.amazon.com/dp/B06WLK7497

http://www.amazon.com/dp/B06W54JKQN
http://www.amazon.com/dp/B06X6DJ9K3
http://www.amazon.com/dp/B06WGNJ9N3
http://www.amazon.com/dp/B06W549TBD
http://www.amazon.com/dp/B06VTF5DQJ
http://www.amazon.com/dp/B06WRPSBKK
http://www.amazon.com/dp/B06WD194JR
http://www.amazon.com/dp/B06WCZTK7Y
http://www.amazon.com/dp/B06X3QN1HT
http://www.amazon.com/dp/B01N19WBF2
http://www.amazon.com/dp/B01N2AVECA
http://www.amazon.com/dp/B01N4VZIAV
http://www.amazon.com/dp/B00QJJFS1C
http://www.amazon.com/dp/B01EMNO2MW
http://www.amazon.com/dp/B00SSFWCPA
http://www.amazon.com/dp/1520531230
http://www.amazon.com/dp/B01N4V7SR9
http://www.amazon.com/dp/B00SX58DUI
http://www.amazon.com/dp/B010K7YP62
http://www.amazon.com/dp/B012LAYNNQ
http://www.amazon.com/dp/B00RVX3KY2
http://www.amazon.com/dp/B01MR6SWGW

http://www.amazon.com/dp/B00XF6G4HO
http://www.amazon.com/dp/B01F1472N2
http://www.amazon.com/dp/B00PQ0TUPU
http://www.amazon.com/dp/B00PP8OZJ4
http://www.amazon.com/dp/B00QH7DY4Y
http://www.amazon.com/dp/B01052010G
http://www.amazon.com/dp/B00QDHXN7Q
http://www.amazon.com/dp/B00PO0IQIO

Among others.

www.ingramcontent.com/pod-product-compliance
Lightning Source LLC
Chambersburg PA
CBHW050929290526
45792CB00002B/937